Anti Inflammatory Diet

Beginners Guide To Avoid Inflammation and Eliminate Pain With Anti-Inflammatory Diet Recipes

Introduction

I want to welcome you to this amazing guide on the anti-inflammatory diet along with quick and easy recipes that you can make to help prevent and reduce your current inflammation.

Inside this book it contains proven steps and strategies on how to eliminate inflammation from your body to help ease pain and live and healthier, happier life.

You may want to read this short book over a few times to let the new knowledge sink in and enjoy the golden nuggets inside like so many other people have.

Let's dive right in!

Chapter 1 – What is Inflammation?

Many of you must have read different medical opinions on what really is inflammation and certainly a lot of those reading these lines have tried to end up the pain with medication not that efficient as initially thought.

This is mainly because inflammation can be caused by various factors and is not always that most popular drugs can help.

Briefly, inflammation is a process by which some particular white cells of the body, also named leukocytes, together with substances they produce, have the function of protecting us from infection with foreign organisms, such as bacteria and viruses. Some individuals will think that this is normal and that inflammation is, therefore, a good sign. Acute inflammation prevents the spread of infectious agents and damage to nearby tissues, helps to remove damaged tissue and pathogens, and assists the body's repair processes.

There are situations in which, as studies proved, inflammation can lead to the development of degenerative diseases, and here we talk about chronic inflammation or silent inflammation, as Dr. Barry Sears, Ph.D. coined it.

This can be triggered by excessive calories consumption and oxidative stress. Stress-induced inflammation is strongly related to aging process.

Autoimmune response is yet another problem that inflammation could possibly represent. The body's defense system identifies an infection when, in fact, there are no foreign anti-corps that are invading the organism. The most common type of such physical affection is arthritis, which can be: rheumatoid, psoriatic or gouty.

Inflammation is able to produce a lot of symptoms which, remember, don't compulsory mean that you have somewhere in your body an inflammation.

From them we remind: redness, swollen joint that's sometimes warm to the touch, joint pain, joint stiffness, loss of joint function.

It can also be associated with general flu-like symptoms like for instance fever, chills, fatigue/loss of energy, headaches, loss of appetite, muscle stiffness.

However, you should notice that inflammation influences the health of your cardiovascular system, affects how quickly your injuries heal and plays a role in determining whether or not you catch a cold.

In order to determine if within your organism there has been settled an inflammation, you should take a blood test which measures two biomarkers linked to the presence of such: c-reactive protein and white blood cells.

C-reactive protein is directly related to the stage of inflammation, while white blood cells in great number don't necessarily prove that you have got an inflammation.

Their role is to fight infections, but their presence is also influenced by stress, trauma, allergies, certain diseases you could have.

Risk factors which increase the likelihood of developing chronic inflammation are closely related to age, obesity and diet, sexual hormones, smoking, sleep disorders, excessive blood glucose.

Studies connect a lot of types of affections with inflammation: allergy, Alzheimer's, anemia, Ankylosing Spondylitis, asthma, autism, arthritis, congestive heart failure, eczema, cardiovascular diseases, cancer, diabetes, macular degeneration (medical condition that usually affects older adults and results in a loss of vision in the center of the visual field, the macula, because of damage to the retina), chronic kidney disease, osteoporosis, depression, cognitive decline, pancreatitis, anemia, fibromyalgia, frailty, muscle wasting, fibrosis, heart attack, lupus, psoriasis, stroke.

It is proven that in some of these affections, inflammation is present in a certain shape, at cellular level or organ-directed level. Some of these are auto-immune diseases.

Cancer is terrifying and it can be connected to inflammation, but we have some good news: keeping under control inflammation can reduce chances that cancer develops. Chronic inflammation creates an ideal environment for free radicals, rogue molecules that travel through the body leaving a path of destruction in their wake. If a healthy cell's DNA is damaged by free radicals, it may mutate. Continuing to grow and divide, it may transform into a cancerous tumor. Therefore, free radicals stimulate the evolution of an inflammation.

Chapter 2 – Foods That Can Cause Inflammation

Not only can food increase the level of the inflammation, but it can add some more chronic conditions such as obesity, diabetes and heart disease.

Let's start with ingredients that can enhance your sufferance: white refined sugar, with the comment that natural carbohydrates are not damaging or saturated fat which can trigger fat tissue inflammation, contained in some kinds of cheese, meat, pasta and grain-based desserts, trans fats, encountered in fried products, processed snack foods, cookies, donuts, stick margarines, fast food.

To the list of substances that can trigger the body to produce pro-inflammatory chemicals we can add: omega 6 acids, found in oils such corn, safflower, sunflower, grape-seed, soy, peanut, refined carbohydrates composing white flour products, white rice, white potatoes, refined cereals products, mono-sodium glutamate , a flavor-enhancing food additive that can be found in soy sauce, different sorts of Asian food, prepared soups, salad dressings, deli meats, affecting the liver. Last, but not least, we should refrain from consuming products containing gluten and casein.

When you are trying to give up sugar in order to lose weight, have you reflected upon the effects the substitutes can have? Aspartame is a neurotoxin and if your body attacks it, then its response will be an inflammatory one.

Let's think about some wild party. Excessive use of alcohol disrupts multi-organ interactions and can cause inflammation.

For how many of you has the thought of being vegetarian or vegan become reality?

Well, you ought to know that meat and poultry tend to cause inflammation, but wild-caught fish can offer you omega 3, minerals and vitamins that protect your organism against chronic inflammation. With the purpose of counteracting inflammation, is important to balance the quantities of omega-3 and omega 6 acids that you ingest. We usually intake a surplus of omega-6 acids from sunflower or corn oil, which you can find in fast food and other processed products, as well as from oil-rich seeds.

Other enemies that contribute to this imbalanced ratio are margarine and partially hydrogenated vegetable oils. Oily fish, walnuts, flax, hemp, and to a lesser degree soy and sea vegetables, contain omega-3 acids.

Getting to the point, vegetarians, vegans or vegetarians that eat only fish as meat not only get more omega-3 acids, but more antioxidants in order to fight free-radicals that get to a high degree of inflammation.

Besides other products written above, dairy ones such as yoghurt, ice-cream, cottage cheese, butter, other kinds of cheese, are very often packed with hormones or antibiotics, so try to avoid them or at least try to identify from where they come and what is the trace of the product, the origin of ingredients and the manner in which the final product is obtained.

Iodized salt is sometimes depleted of its natural minerals with only sodium left or is refined using harmful substances as heavy metals or anti-caking additives that are not healthy.

Reading this gets you thinking that you will have to eliminate more than 50 percent of what you are usually eating? Don't worry, red meat, fat and carbohydrates are not so bad if they originate from natural, ecological or bio sources. Small producers still give attention to what they put in the food.

If you cannot afford them all the time, then at least you can be attentive to the way you mix different types of food when you consume them.

Substances and aliments proved to be efficient in curing and preventing inflammation-related diseases: ginger, melatonin, green leafs, resveratrol, vitamin D, zinc, magnesium, Gotu Kola – a herb, green tea, forest berries, papaya, turmeric, rosemary,

Sedentary lifestyle is another risk factor that can foster the development of chronic inflammation. Studies have shown that constant and not effort-exaggerated physical exercises can prevent diseases associated with it.

Chapter 3 – Anti-Inflammatory Breakfast Recipes

(Quick & Simple) Oatmeal porridge:

Ingredients:

- 1 cup of water
- ½ cup dry quinoa
- ½ cup dry unsweetened cherries
- ½ teaspoon vanilla extract
- ¼ teaspoon ground cinnamon
- 1 tablespoon honey (optional)
-

Mix 1 cup of water with ½ cup dry quinoa, ½ cup dry unsweetened cherries (contain anthocyanin which fights with inflammation), ½ teaspoon vanilla extract, ¼ teaspoon ground cinnamon and, optionally, 1 tablespoon honey (optional) – boil the first five ingredients at medium-high heat, then reduce heat until all the water has been absorbed

Anti-inflammatory juice:

Ingredients:

- 2 roots of celery
- ½ small pineapple
- 1 small cucumber
- ¼ lemon
- ½ fresh ginger

Cut in small pieces and blend together 2 roots of celery, ½ small pineapple, 1 small cucumber, ¼ lemon, ½ fresh ginger

Anti-inflammatory smoothie:

Ingredients:

- 2 parts pineapple
- 1 part mango
- 1 piece of ginger
- ½ part of celery
- 1 part coconut water
- 1 teaspoon of vanilla

This quick smoothie is easy to whip up fast and is super healthy!

All you need to do is mix all ingredients in a blender and blend then you're done.

Poached Eggs with Curried Vegetables:

Ingredients:

- 2 teaspoons extra-virgin olive oil
- 1 large chopped onion
- 2 minced cloves of garlic
- 1 tablespoon yellow curry powder
- ½ pound sliced button mushrooms
- 2 medium diced zucchinis
- 1 14-ounce can drained chickpeas
- ⅛ teaspoon of crushed red pepper (optional)
- 1 cup of water
- ½ teaspoon of white vinegar
- 4 large eggs

On a medium to high heat sauté onions until they become mild, then add garlic and cook for 30 seconds; stir in curry powder and cook 1-2 minutes; continue by adding mushrooms and cook until they release their liquid (~ 5 minutes); afterwards, add the zucchini, the chickpeas, the water and, optionally, some red pepper, then boil everything; reduce heat and simmer covered, for 15-20 minutes.

Omelet with spinach and goat cheese:

Ingredients:

- Goat cheese (how much you like)
- Butter (enough to coat pan)
- Black pepper and salt
- Herbs (parsley chives, tarragon
- 1 handful of baby spinach
- 2 tablespoon coconut milk
- 3 eggs

This is a gluten-free recipe, full of fresh spices.

You will need goat cheese, butter, black pepper, sea salt, fresh herbs parsley chives, tarragon, 1 handful of baby spinach, 2 tablespoons of sour cream or coconut milk, 1 egg, lettuce. Before preparation, it is a good idea to soak the eggs in tap water, in order to bring them to room temperature and help them cook more easily.

In the meantime you can chop the herbs and spinach. Eggs are then combined with salt, pepper, milk and then well mixed together. Melt the butter at medium heat and spread it well in the pan.

When it starts to take on a brownish hue, add the egg mixture and greens. Cook for about 1-2 minutes, until bake well. Put the omelet on a plate and fill it with lettuce and cheese. From this meal you'll receive all the necessary nutrients without having to worry for later inflammations.

Chapter 4 – Delicious Anti-Inflammatory Lunch Recipes

Pumpkin Soup

Ingredients

- 1 cup chopped onion
- 1 1-inch piece gingerroot, peeled and minced
- 1 clove garlic, minced
- 6 cups vegetable stock, divided
- 4 cups pumpkin puree
- 1 teaspoon salt
- ½ teaspoon chopped fresh thyme
- ½ cup half-and-half
- 1 teaspoon chopped fresh parsley

Preparation: Cook onions, garlic and ginger in ½ cup vegetable stock, about 5 minutes. Then add pumpkin, the remaining 5 ½ cups stock, pour some salt and thyme and cook for 30 minutes. Mix in the blender all the ingredients. You can serve it with chopped parsley.

Pumpkin is full of carotenoids, antioxidants which absorb free radicals that attack the body and protects it from disease, strengthening the immunity. Beta-carotene in pumpkin fights effectively against inflammatory diseases of the skin and lungs.

White Bean and Chicken Chili Blanca

Ingredients

- 1 pound chicken tenders or boneless, skinless chicken breasts

- 2 tablespoons of extra-virgin olive oil

- 1 medium diced onion

- 2 garlic cloves

- 2 15-ounce cans of white or great northern beans, drained and rinsed

- 1 cup corn kernels, fresh or frozen and thawed

- 1 4-ounce can chopped green chilies

- 2 teaspoons of ground cumin

- 2 teaspoons of pure chilies powder

- 1/8 teaspoon of cayenne pepper

- 3 cups of water

- 2 cups grated Monterey Jack cheese

- 2 tablespoons chopped fresh cilantro

Preparation: season the chicken with salt and pepper; then, in a large saucepan, heat oil over high heat, add chicken pieces and cook for 2-3 minutes; afterwards, lower the heat to medium, add onion and garlic and cook until the onion is translucent, let's say about 5-6 minutes; after this, add the beans, corn, chilies, spices and water; bring to a boil, reduce heat to low and simmer uncovered for 1 hour; optionally, you can top each serving with a spoonful of cheese and sprinkling of cilantro.

White beans are abundant in fiber, thereby minimizing the risk of heart disease, improving bowel function, maintaining a feeling of satiety for a long time. A special kind of fiber contained in beans is responsible for a mild increase in blood glucose levels, important for diabetics and people who want to lose weight.

Fibers contained in the beans, without any caloric intake, also reduce the level of harmful cholesterol in the body.

Overall, vegetable fibers beans prevent the absorption of sugars and reduce insulin secretion.

Baked Salmon

Ingredients:

- 150 g salmon fillet
- 3 tablespoons of olive oil
- 3 cherry tomatoes
- 5 tablespoons of water
- 1 tablespoon of sliced olives
- half a lemon juice
- salt and pepper to taste

Preparation: in a bowl of Jena baking paper is put; the paper must be on all the vessel walls; the salmon is added after which salt, pepper, tomatoes (cut into 4 pieces), oil, water, olives, olive oil and the lemon juice are poured over and around, soaking the meat; it is important to note that the oven should be preheated; everything inside the bowl needs to be covered with paper from the sidelines and baked for 20-30 minutes on low heat.

Salmon is a type of fish with an increased content of omega 3 fatty acids, essential nutrients in controlling inflammation in the body. It seems that Alaska wild salmon is the most powerful anti-inflammatory kind of meat and contains substances that are calming for the body.

Chicken with shiitake mushrooms

Ingredients:

- 1 chicken breast
- 1 red bell pepper
- 6 fresh shiitake mushrooms

- 1 green onion thread
- 2 cloves garlic
- 3 tablespoons vegetable oil
- 3 tablespoons soy sauce
- 1 teaspoon rice wine (cooking alcohol)
- 1 teaspoon sugar
- 1/3 teaspoon salt
- 2 teaspoons starch

Preparation: Cut the chicken breasts into thin strips, placed in a bowl; over it put 1 tablespoon of soy sauce, pour the rice wine, add 1 teaspoon starch and 1 pinch of salt.; allow the whole compound to marinate for 20 minutes.

In the meanwhile we slice the vegetables down (red peppers cut into thin strips, shiitake mushrooms in larger strips, sliced onions and garlic finely chopped); if you do not have fresh shiitake mushrooms, dried mushrooms can be used without problems after being rehydrated for half an hour in warm water.

In a pan we heat up 2 tablespoons of vegetable oil and fry the chicken strips until they crisp easy and get a nice golden color; we remove the chicken from the pan and leave it aside; we place again the pan in heat, pour the remaining oil, add garlic and onions, pepper, shiitake mushrooms and fry for more than two minutes; we mix all well and pour soy sauce over; starch is dissolved in 2 tablespoons of cold water and poured; we mix a few seconds slowly until the sauce thickens; we garnish with green onions after.

Mushrooms are not only a rich source of protein for your health, but also a source of antioxidants and nutrients that fight effectively against inflammation in the body. Shiitake mushrooms are the species with the most powerful anti-inflammatory effects.

Mashed sweet potatoes with chicken and coconut ginger sauce

Ingredients:

- 2 large sweet potatoes

- 6 boneless chicken thighs
- soy sauce
- orange flower water
- coconut powder
- ginger
- orange blossom water
- 1 garlic
- milk
- butter

Preparation: The 6 boneless chicken thighs are marinated for a day in a mixture made from soy sauce, orange flower water, curry, chilly, and dry basil; after the process they are cut in very thin slices, covered in eggs and sprinkled with sesame; the slices are fried in oil; while the chicken is prepared, we boil the sweet potatoes; after the potatoes have boiled they are put in a blender with garlic, butter and milk; milk can be further added to the mixture until the desired consistency is obtained; a special sauce is made from coconut, ginger and orange blossom water.

Sweet potato is a rich source of carbohydrates, beta-carotene, fiber, manganese and vitamins B and C. All of these nutrients in potato fight effectively against inflammation in the body and combat with efficiency any form of physical pain.

Chapter 5 – Tastiest Anti-Inflammatory Dessert Recipes

Raw Truffles with Mint and Coffee

Ingredients:

- 2 cans of dates
- 2 cans of nuts
- 2 tablespoons of raw cocoa
- ½ can of fresh mint
- 1 shot of espresso
- 1 pinch of Himalaya salt
- ½ glass of cocoa beans

Put the nuts into the blender and grain them, add the cocoa and the salt and homogenize everything.

While the blender is on, put inside the coffee shot, the mint and the dates and mix until the whole ingredients become one. Put the composition into the fridge and let it there for 30 minutes.

Fruit salad with anti-inflammatory properties

Ingredients:

- Small fruit papaya

- Half a fresh pineapple

- 400 grams mix of berries (blackberries, blueberries, raspberries, strawberries)

- 1 sliced apple

- Juice from one lemon

- Juice from one orange

- Handful of chopped almonds

- 1 tablespoon honey (optional)

We will need a small fruit papaya, peeled and diced, half a fresh pineapple, peeled and chopped, 400 grams mix of berries (blackberries, blueberries, raspberries, strawberries, etc.), 1 sliced apple, shell and juice from one lemon, juice from one orange, a handful of chopped almonds, 1 tablespoon honey (optional).

We mix in a small bowl the lemon, citrus juice and honey. In another large bowl, we add the cubes of papaya, pineapple, berries and apple slices. We pour over the dressing obtained in the small bowl and mix gently so that all fruits are well covered. Last, we garnish the salad with chopped almonds. The anti-inflammatory effect is guaranteed by the presence of almonds and papaya.

Caramelized apples with fried walnuts

Ingredients:

- 40g walnuts (chopped)
- 40 g sugar (stevia)
- 2 tablespoons water
- ¼ teaspoon ground nutmeg
- 4 large golden apples

This is a dessert which can be ready in around 20 minutes.

We will need 40g walnuts, chopped, 40-50 g stevia (sugar sweetener), 2 tablespoons water, ¼ teaspoon ground nutmeg, 4 large golden apples, peeled and sliced and natural yogurt for serving.

The nuts are fried in a medium skillet over moderate heat for 3-4 minutes until they become slightly browned. Then they are removed from the pan and put aside.

We combine the sugar sweetener, water and nutmeg in the pan, reduce heat to minimum and stir frequently until sugar melts and bubbles out.

We then add the apple slices in the pan. We stir until the slices are "dressed" in caramelized sugar. We further cook until the apples become tender. We sprinkle over the walnuts and place in bowls. The dessert is served with natural yoghurt.

Cookies with oatmeal and raisins

This is a dessert which can be ready in around 15 minutes. We will need as ingredients the following: 75g brown or white sugar, 50 g of granulated sugar, 150 ml of applesauce, 1 large egg, 80 ml of skimmed milk, 1 teaspoon vanilla, 340 g of flour with increasing agent (or mixed with 1 teaspoon tip of baking powder, ½ teaspoon nutmeg, 340 g of oatmeal, 150 g of raisins. The oven is preheated to 190 degrees C. We mix the sugar and applesauce, add egg and beat well. We then add milk and vanilla, then flour and beat well. Add the remaining ingredients together and blend. The mixture is well spread on tray with a baking sheet on, putting each tablespoon at a distance of 2-3 cm apart from the others. The tray is then inserted in the oven and kept for about 9 minutes until the cookies become crisp.

- **Dietetic brownies with bananas**

  A brownie should not be a forbidden fruit for those who are on a strict diet that banes certain food, especially desserts. The following ingredients are needed for this recipe: 2 egg whites, 1 teaspoon vanilla, 1/4 teaspoon salt, 1/2 teaspoon baking soda, 1 teaspoon cinnamon, 35g cocoa powder, 70ml buttermilk or weak yogurt, 120g sweetener, 110g buckwheat flour, 180g dark chocolate, 1 large banana sliced. First we mix all dry ingredients: chopped chocolate into small pieces, buckwheat flour, sweetener, cocoa, cinnamon, baking soda and salt. We then make a hole in the middle, where future ingredients will come. We beat the egg, add buttermilk and vanilla. Pour this mixture all at once, inside the hole made in the dry ingredients. Everything is mixed well with a spatula to incorporate ingredients one in each other. We grease a round tray (diameter 20-23cm), pour the compound and arrange the slices of banana on the surface. Everything is covered with aluminum foil and baked in the oven at 160C-170C. The foil should be removed halfway through baking. The dessert it's done when edges begin to detach easily from the pan walls. Let it cool for 30 minutes and you could serve the cake warm.

2 Bonus Recipes That The Whole Family Love
Sweet Potato "Fries"

Give these super healthy sweet potato fries a go and you won't be disappointed!

For the ingredients you'll need:

- 3 unpeeled sweet potatoes or yams, (slice into even strips)
- 1 teaspoon olive oil
- Sea salt and pepper to taste
- Dash of thyme
- Dash of nutmeg

Start by preheating your oven to 400° F.

Drop in a little olive oil with the sweet potatoes, sea salt, and pepper in a nice large bowl to mix.

The next step is to transfer to a baking pan, and then shake over with your nutmeg and thyme seasonings, and then bake for around 30–35 minutes or until the sweet potato is tender enough.

This dish serves 4.

Zucchini Bread

Bread tends to be a staple diet in many household, so rather than eating the typical unhealthy bread that you'll buy from the local grocery store, give this delicious zucchini bread a go.

For the ingredients you'll need:

- ¾ cup organic coconut oil, warmed to liquid consistency
- 3 organic eggs, beaten

- 2 cups grated zucchini
- 1 cup raw honey
- 1 teaspoon vanilla extract
- 3 cups oat flour
- 1 teaspoon baking soda
- ½ teaspoon sea salt

Start by preheating oven to 350° F.

First step is to mix together all wet ingredients plus including the zucchini too.

Slowly start to add the dry ingredients, and mix thoroughly together.

Next step is to pour your batter into a greased 9 x 4 x 3-inch loaf pan.

Finally bake for approx 1 hour or until you can insert a knife in the center and it comes out clean.

This bread serves around 10 slices.

Conclusion

I hope most of all you start taking action on the simple steps to help you to beat inflammation once and for all!

Now even if you apply just a few of the simple tips I've given you today you'll start seeing a massive improvement in your life!

Don't get overwhelmed with all the information and recipes I've given you today, but instead start implementing small changes in your life which what you have learned and over time you will make a bigger momentum shift in your life.

I would also make sure you starting writing down you health and fitness goals. So many people I speak to who don't have goals is crazy. Don't be one them, so start writing down your goals and you will understand exactly where you are heading in life.

Finally, if you enjoyed this book, then I'd like to ask you for a favor, would you be kind enough to leave a review for this book on Amazon? It'd be greatly appreciated!

Thank you and good luck!

Kathy Hunt

Mason Jar Meals

The Tastiest Quick and Easy Mason Jar Recipes On Earth!

By Kathy Hunt

Contents

Introduction

Welcome to the world of mason jar meals and I first want to start off to thank you and congratulate you for downloading the book, Mason *Jar Meals: The Tastiest Quick & Easy Mason Jar Recipes on Earth.*

This book contains proven steps on how I've learned over the years to make delicious, quick, and easy Mason jar meals.

You're going to love the variety and simplicity of these great recipes. Yum!

What's great about the book is that within the next 30 minutes of reading this short and effective Mason jar meals guide you can start taking action right away on which meals tickle your taste buds best!

Let's jump right in!

The Setup for your Mason jar meals

Making your own mason jar meals is not only a great way to be eco-friendly but it is also a great way to prepare meals for a few days to a week in advance. If you plan ahead, you won't have to worry about being too tired or wonder what to make for dinner. Food preparation time is also cut down by using mason jars. Instead of spending a whole weekend cooking food for a month or so and freezing it, you'll only be cooking for a few hours and then you're done!

Mason jars come in all sizes so if you don't want to work with a large jar you can use a small one. The smaller ones also work wonderfully for holding small items such as dressing or shredded cheese.

Other benefits of mason jar meals include

- No more wasted food

- A less cluttered refrigerator

- Not having to worry about what to have for dinner

- No more eating out every day and wondering if it's healthy

- Saves you money

- No more wondering what to do if you're too tired to cook

- Proportion control

There are some great benefits to using mason jars

- Reusable

- Dishwasher safe

- Clear

- Stain proof

- Inexpensive

- Stackable

- Packable

- Microwavable

- Lids can be purchased and reused

You can even freeze some of your meals! Check ahead of time to make sure the food you have packed inside the mason jars are freezer safe. If they are, you can freeze them until you are ready to use them. Not only will you feel good about helping the environment you will also be putting those mason jars to use.

For many occasions, all you have to do is grab a jar, give it a good shake, and enjoy your healthy meal!

Mason jar meals and ideas are popping up all over the news and on blogs. People are even discovering and creating their own recipes to share with the world. Why not join the fun and make your own mason jar meals?

Getting the best results with your mason jar meals

Before you get started on your mason jar meals, you will want to purchase all that you plan on putting into them and clean the food properly. Wash your mason jars with warm soapy water to get rid of any dirt that may be inside of them.

To cook your vegetables, try cutting them into uniform sizes and placing them all in one big pan to cook. You can season your vegetables to taste before putting them in the pan. Doing this will not only save you space, but it will save you time so you do not have to cook everything separate. Set your timer ahead of time so you know which vegetables need to be removed first.

You can cook your meats in the same fashion. Cooking them together will not harm them as long as you cook them properly and for the correct amount of time.

If you have the room in your kitchen, you can multi-task. You can fry bacon, boil your grains and/or pastas, and hard boil your eggs while your meats and vegetables are cooking.

All your items need to be cooked before you place them inside the jars. If you don't do this, your foods can become mushy or not taste very good. If any food came out of the oven, set it aside to cool before placing it inside your jars.

For some foods like oatmeal, it is fairly easy to prepare. You would make your oatmeal like you would any meal, pour it into your mason jar, screw on the lid tightly and leave it to sit until you're ready for it. When you're ready for your oatmeal, you can season it to taste or add in fruits and whatever else you wish to add.

If you don't have the time or feel like you can cook, there are even no cooking options available to you! You can make a fruit yogurt to go. The process is also quite simple as it is only layers. Start by layering your favorite fruit or jam followed by a layer of organic plain yogurt. You can add granola or anything else you would like to each layer and continue until the jar is full.

Before you get started on making some delicious mason jar meals, you will want to decide on what size jars you want to use for each meal. Smaller meals such as yogurt and oatmeal can be held in smaller jars that you can put in your bag or carry with you. For salads and bigger meals such as dinner, you can use bigger jars. It may take some experimenting around to find out what works for you, but the rewards are well worth it.

Even if you feel like you can't cook to save your life, there are many no cook options for breakfast and even deserts available for you so you are never left out!

Amazing "No Cook" Mason Jar Meals

For this chapter I wish to share some no cook mason jar meal options for you. These are fairly simple and can be made in one night and stored for tomorrow.

No cook oatmeal

Ingredients

- One cup steel cut oats
- One scoop protein powder
- One half of an apple of your choice
- Two tablespoons of organic cinnamon
- Fat free skim milk
- One tablespoon cardamom (optional)

Cut your apple into small and uniform pieces.

Add to the mason jar with the steel cut oats, protein powder, and organic cinnamon.

Fill the jar with the skim milk.

Cover and shake well.

Place the full jar in your refrigerator and leave it there over night.

Single serve no bake cheesecake

Ingredients

- Four ½ pint mason jars

- One 8oz packaged cream cheese

- 1 can (14oz) sweetened condensed milk

- Two tablespoons lemon juice (this can be modified according to taste)

- One teaspoon vanilla extract

- Your choice of toppings

- Graham crackers for crust.

Follow the directions on your favorite recipe for the gram cracker crust.

Mix cream cheese, juice and condensed milk until creamy and smooth.

Pour this onto the prepared crust and top with topping of choice.

Place inside your refrigerator and let chill for at least three hours.

Wheat berry apple salad

Ingredients

- Three cups cooked wheat berries

- One half granny smith apple, chopped

- One-third cup dried cranberries

- One scallion, minced

- Two tablespoons parsley, chopped

- One tablespoon lemon juice

- One tablespoon balsamic vinegar

- One half tablespoon olive oil

Mix wheat berries, granny smith apple, cranberries, scallion, and parsley in a bowl and set aside.

Whisk the lemon juice, balsamic vinegar, and olive oil until well combined.

Mix with salad and toss well.

Serves four.

Tasty Breakfast Jars Meals

If you wish to try for other tasty breakfast meals these will work wonderfully. It's best to prepare them a night or two before you plan to eat them so they're still fresh.

Oven baked egg and vegetable cups

Ingredients

- Six to seven half pint mason jars

- Two teaspoons olive oil

- One half large onion

- One bundle of asparagus

- Ten eggs, beaten

- Three-fourths cup grated cheese

- Salt

- Pepper

Instructions

Preheat your oven to 375 degrees.

Cut the large onion into thin half-moons. Wash the asparagus well and trim the ends. Cut the asparagus into chunks from ½ to ¾ inches wide.

Heat some oil in a large skillet and add the onions. Cook these until brown.

Add the asparagus chunks and cook until a tender crisp. This should take roughly five minutes. Season to taste with salt and pepper and set aside.

Grease the mason jars. Using tongs portion out the sautéed vegetables into the jars. They should be mostly filled with vegetables.

Beat the eggs and evenly divide them into the jars.

Top with approximately one tablespoon of cheese per jar. Using a fork carefully stir the contents of each jar so the cheese just isn't sitting on the top.

Place the jars on a baking sheet and bake for 20 to 25 minutes. When the tops are browned they are done.

Once removed from the oven let them cool. You can place lids on the jars once they are cool to the touch.

Store the egg vegetable cups in the refrigerator until ready to eat. They will keep for up to five days.

Blueberry French toast

Ingredients

- One third loaf of bread

- One tablespoon vanilla

- One tablespoon cinnamon

- One fourth cup sugar

- One and a half cups milk

- Two eggs

- Blueberries (as many as desired)

- Two tablespoons melted butter

- One fourth cup maple syrup

Instructions

Cut loaf of bread into cubes and place in jars

Combine milk, eggs, vanilla, sugar, cinnamon, blueberries, syrup, and butter into a mixing bowl and hand mix well before pouring evening into jars.

Cover the jars and store upside down in your refrigerator overnight.

Heat your oven to 375 degrees and cook jars **uncovered** for 45 minutes or until top is a golden brown.

Once cool top with maple syrup.

Nutella breakfast

Ingredients

- Half pint mason jar

- One tablespoon Nutella

- One-fourth cup oatmeal

- One half cup almond milk

- Strawberries

- Yogurt (Optional)

Instructions

Combine oatmeal, almond milk and Nutella. Mix ingredients until Nutella is completely integrated. This mixture should look light brown.

Top with your strawberries and refrigerate overnight.

Lunch Meals "On the Go"

There are many good options out there for lunch on the go. Making your own mason jar meals for lunch is a great option. You won't have to worry about going out to lunch or not having money for lunch. Your meal will be right there in the building and you'll know what you paid for.

Some delicious recipes include

Chicken Ramen Salad

Ingredients

- One pound bag of shredded cabbage

- Three green onions, sliced

- Three handfuls slivered almonds

- One can of Mandarin oranges, drained

- Two cups pre-cooked chicken, chopped

- One package oriental flavored ramen noodles

- One third cup rice vinegar

- One third cup sugar

- One half cup vegetable oil

- Sesame seeds for garnish (optional)

Instructions

In a large bowl mix shredded cabbage, onions, almonds, Mandarin oranges, and chicken and toss.

Crush the ramen noodles but **only** before eating to prevent sogginess.

Using a blender blend vinegar, sugar, oil, and seasoning packet from ramen noodles. You can serve the dressing on the side or toss it with the salad.

Garnish with sesame seeds.

Will serve six.

Sushi in a jar

Ingredients

- Three fourths cup cooked short grain brown rice

- One tablespoon rice vinegar (if you're using seasoned rice vinegar ignore the sugar and heat)

- One teaspoon sugar

- One to two teaspoons soy sauce

- One sheet nori, cut into one by one-fourth inch pieces

- One fourth cup shredded carrot

- One fourth cup cucumber matchsticks

- One half an avocado, diced

- Lime juice

- Pickled ginger (to taste)

- Wasabi paste (to taste)

Instructions

Heat the vinegar and sugar in a small saucepan over medium heat until the sugar is dissolved. (If you used season rice vinegar ignore this step.)

While the brown rice is warm pour the vinegar-sugar mix and soy sauce over it and toss. Let it cool to room temperature.

When you prepare your vegetables place the diced avocado in a bowl and toss with just enough lime juice to lightly coat it to prevent browning.

Once your ingredients are prepared add them to your jar one at a time using a spoon. The order which you choose to add them is entirely up to you. After finishing with one layer gently pat it down with your spoon and begin the next.

Gazpacho in a Jar

Ingredients

- One large mason jar
- Tomato juice
- Four parts tomatoes, diced
- Two parts cucumber, diced
- One part bell pepper, diced
- One half part thinly sliced green onions
- One half part extra virgin olive oil
- One handful cilantro leaves
- A few cloves of garlic
- Your favorite seasonings (optional)

Instructions

Mix ingredients thoroughly in a blender and pour into jar.

Place in refrigerator and allow to chill.

If you wish to make this later or give this as a gift arrange everything in nice layers with a note on what to do.

Easy (no fuss) Quick Dinners

Mason jar meals aren't just for breakfast and lunches. You can also make tasty easy to make recipes for dinner and even deserts. Yum!

Dinner rolls in a jar

Ingredients

- Small mason jars

- One fourth cup butter

- One teaspoon salt

- One fourth cup water

- One cup milk

- One fourth cup sugar

- One teaspoon yeast

- One egg, beaten

- Four to five cups flour

- One tablespoon butter, melted

- One fourth teaspoon fresh garlic, finely minced

- One fourth dried rosemary

Instructions

Preheat your oven to 375 degrees.

Heat the milk, butter, salt, water, and sugar in a small saucepan on the stove over a **medium heat** until sugar is dissolved.

Pour mixture into a mixing bowl and add yeast, eggs, and two cups of flower and mix well. Start adding one half cup of flour at a time to make for soft dough and mix for one minute.

Place mixture into large greased bowl and let rise until doubled in size.

Place jars on a cookie sheet and spray with a non-stick cooking spray.

After dough has risen form balls of dough and place one in each jar. Each boll of dough should fill up half the jar. Let rise again until it has doubled in size.

In small bowl, mix butter, garlic, and rosemary. Brush butter mixture on top of each roll.

Bake for 18-20 minutes or until lightly browned.

Easy Spanish rice

Ingredients

- One large jar of Ragu Green Pepper sauce

- Two bags of minute rice (brown rice works well too)

- One pound lean ground beef

Instructions

Preheat oven to 375 degrees

Cook the rice according to the directions written on the package.

In a large baking pan mix cooked rice, jar of sauce, and uncooked crumbled beef.

Bake uncovered for one hour and place in large jars for your next meal.

Chicken pot pies in jars

Ingredients

- Dough for a double pie crust (homemade or store-bought is fine.)

- Two tablespoons of butter and two teaspoons of butter, cut and divided

- One half medium onion, diced

- Three medium carrots, diced

- One cup cooked chicken, diced

- Two cups milk

- One cup chicken broth

- Two to three tablespoons flour

- One half cup frozen peas

- Salt and pepper

Instructions

Preheat your oven to 425 degrees.

Using **medium heat** melt **two teaspoons** butter and sauté carrots until lightly cooked. This should take two to three minutes. Add the onions and cook for an additional two minutes. When this is done set the pan aside.

In a large saucepan using **medium heat** melt the remaining **two tablespoons** of butter and then add two to three tablespoons of flour and cook for one to two minutes until the mixture is lightly browned. This is going to be a paste like mixture.

Whisk in the milk and broth one cup at a time. You will bring each cup to a boil before adding the next cup.

Add chicken and pea, and then simmer for five to seven minutes until sauce has thickened.

Roll out the pie crusts and cut each of them into quarters. Line each jar with the crust making sure all the edges are sealed.

Scoop the filling into the jars and then roll out the remaining pie crust to top the jars. Use a fork to seal around the edges.

Bake the jars for fifteen minutes until crust has lightly browned. Remove the pies from the oven to cover with foil and bake for another fifteen minutes.

My Favorite Cake Jar Recipe

S'mores Cake in a Jar

Ingredients

Crust

- One and a half cups graham cracker crumbs
- One half stick butter
- Pinch of salt
- Preheat oven to 350 degrees.

Cake

- One and one-eighth cups all-purpose flour
- One fourth cup dark cocoa powder
- One and one fourth teaspoon baking soda
- One half teaspoon salt
- Three-fourths cup brown sugar
- One egg
- One teaspoon vanilla extract
- One half cup milk

- One half cup and one tablespoon heavy cream

- One half cup butter, melted

- Two tablespoons sour cream

- One bag marshmallows

Instructions

Preheat your oven to 350 degrees.

Melt the butter and mix in graham crumbs and salt. Mix until it is moistened.

Spray four mason jars with non-stick cooking spray and press gram cracker crumbs into jars.

In a bowl whisk the egg and sugar until smooth and there are no lumps. Add milk, cream, butter, vanilla and mix until well combined. Stir in the sour cream.

Sift dry ingredients together and add to the wet mixture. Mix until the batter is smooth.

Using a one-fourth cup measure and add batter to the mason jars one scoop at a time. You only want to find them up to about half way.

Place jars in a baking dish and add one and a half cups water at the bottom.

Bake for 30 minutes.

Remove cake from the oven and press large marshmallows down on top. Be careful not to burn yourself!

Heat the broiler on your oven and brown the marshmallows for one to two minutes. These can burn very quickly so be careful when using the broiler!

Taking action on my mason jar meals

Thank you again for downloading this book!

Making Mason jar meals is very easy and a great way to keep on top of things.

There are many more delicious recipes online at your fingertips. You can join a message board, start a blog, and connect with other people who are also making Mason jar meals!

Have fun and enjoy!

Finally, if you enjoyed this book, then I'd like to ask you for a favor, would you be kind enough to leave a review for this book on Amazon? It'd be greatly appreciated!

Click here to leave a review for this book on Amazon!

Thank you and good luck!

Mason Jar Lunches

Quick and Easy Lunch Time Jar Recipes

By Kathy Hunt

Contents

Introduction

Welcome to this beginners recipe guide on mason jar lunches, where you will discover how to create amazing mason jar lunches quick and easy without the fuss.

Once you start using these mason jar lunch recipes you will soon see why mason jar lunches are becoming so popular worldwide.

If you want to save your time making lunches and save a bit of extra cash then these mason jar salads will blown your mind (not to forget they are incredibly tasty too).

Inside I will teach you the little known tips and tricks to get the best results from your mason jar lunches and will give you many options to now tickle your taste buds every lunch time.

Enjoy!

Kathy Hunt

Chapter 1 – Tasty Chicken Lunch Recipes

Chicken is very versatile and works great for lunches. It packs quite easily into a mason jar and you can make any of these easy and tasty recipes!

Greek Salad

If you like Greek salads this a great one to try. It is filled with tomatoes, cucumbers, chicken, and more! Best of all you can even customize it to your own tastes. This particular recipe contains enough salad to fill five quart sized mason jars. You can adjust the recipe as needed and for taste. Unless you wish for a marinated salad put the dressing on the bottom.

Ingredients

- Five quart size wide mouth mason jars
- Ten tablespoons your favorite salad dressing

- One quart cherry tomatoes, halved

- Five mini cucumbers, sliced

- One cup pitted Greek olives, sliced or chopped

- Three fourths cup crumbled feta cheese

- Two cups chopped or shredded rotisserie chicken

- Five cups chopped romaine lettuce

Instructions

Separate and layer all ingredients into your mason jars. Start by pouring the salad dressing first. By pouring the salad dressing first nothing can get soggy. Place tomatoes on top of the salad dressing followed by the cucumbers, olives, cheese, chicken, and top with lettuce.

Place the lid on top of the mason jar and store in the refrigerator until ready to eat.

Grilled Chicken Salad

Do you still want to try a salad but don't like Greek salad? There's no need to worry because I've got you covered! Why not try this tasty grilled chicken salad? Unless you wish for a marinated salad put the dressing on the bottom.

Ingredients

- Six ounce boneless chicken breast
- Lettuce
- One hard-boiled egg
- Two ounces bacon
- Eight croutons
- Three tomato wedges
- Marinade
- One half pound brown sugar
- One cup soy sauce
- One cup sherry
- Three cups pineapple juice

- One half cup red wine vinegar
- One teaspoon granulated garlic
- One half teaspoon ground ginger
- Vinaigrette
- One cup cotton seed oil
- One cup red wine vinegar
- One fourth garlic clove
- One teaspoon salt
- One teaspoon black pepper
- One teaspoon crushed oregano
- One fourth cup sugar
- One fourth cup Dijon mustard

Instructions

Marinade: in a large bowl combine brown sugar, soy sauce, sherry, pineapple juice, vinegar, garlic, and ginger. Mix well and set aside. This will make enough marinate for about six chicken breasts.

Vinaigrette: in a blender combine oil, vinegar, garlic, salt, pepper, oregano, sugar, and mustard. Mix well until fully blended and set aside.

Prepare the marinade and marinate the chicken, skin side up, for at least three hours. After the three hours have passed grill the chicken and remove the skin. Discard the skin as you do not need it.

Inside a mason jar pour the vinaigrette dressing first. Place the tomato wedges on top followed by the egg, bacon, chicken, lettuce. Set the croutons aside until you are ready to eat your salad.

Place the lid on the mason jar and refrigerate until ready to eat.

Chicken Noodle Soup in a Jar

Who doesn't like soup during those cold winter days? This is a simple and easy way to make chicken noodle soup to bring with you for lunch.

Ingredients

- One cup egg noodles (uncooked fine)
- One and one half tablespoons chicken bouillon granules
- One half teaspoon ground black pepper
- One fourth teaspoon thyme (dried whole)
- One eighth teaspoon celery seed
- One eighth teaspoon garlic powder
- One bay leaf
- Two carrots (diced)
- Two celery ribs (diced)
- One fourth cup minced onion
- Three cups cooked chicken

Instructions

In a large stock pot combine the noodles, chicken bouillon, black pepper, thyme, celery, garlic, bay leaf and eight cups of water. Add two diced carrots, two stalks of diced celery, and one fourth cup minced onion.

Bring the mixture to a boil. Cover the soup and reduce the heat to a simmer and let simmer for fifteen minutes.

Discard the bay leaf.

Stir in three cups of diced chicken and let simmer for five minutes.

Season to taste.

Once everything is cooked and cooled sufficiently spoon the soup into mason jars and close the lids. These can easily be warmed up at work for a hearty soup.

Mesquite Chicken

If you have any leftover chicken this is a tasty way to make yourself a good lunch and so that nothing goes to waste!

Ingredients

- Four boneless chicken breasts
- One large can pineapple chunks
- One jar broiled mushroom pieces (or fresh mushrooms sliced and sautéed in butter)
- One pound deli sliced honey ham
- Four thick slices of Monterey Jack cheese
- Twelve ounces mesquite cooking sauce and marinade

Instructions

In a large skillet mix the pineapples with their juices and add the chicken breasts. Cook over a medium-high heat until the breasts are no longer pink in the middle. Remove the meat from the skillet and discard any juices.

Cut up and place the chicken inside a mason jar. On top of that pour the mesquite marinade all over the pieces. Add the mushrooms and then the ham. If you plan on eating it right away put the cheese on top of each chicken piece. If not, save the cheese until you are ready to eat. You can warm it up by cooking everything for about two minutes on the high setting on your microwave.

Chapter 2 – Beautiful Beef Lunch Recipes On the Go

If you tire of chicken why not try some great tasting beef recipes? Here I'll be listing four great and easy to do recipes that you can have on the go!

Beef Stew

Who doesn't like a hearty beef stew on a cold day?

Ingredients

- Two to two and a half pounds beef stew meat, cut into one and a half inch cubes

- One and one half teaspoon vegetable oil

- Six cups cubed and peeled potatoes

- Four cups sliced carrots

- One and one half cups chopped celery

- One and one half cups chopped onion

- Three fourths teaspoon salt

- One half teaspoon thyme

- One fourth teaspoon pepper

- Water

- Three quart sized mason jars

Instructions

Brown the beef in oil and in a large skillet. Once the meat is browned and not pink in the middle transfer the meat into a large sauce pot and discard the liquid via your preferred method.

Add the vegetables and seasoning.

Cover in water and bring stew to a boil.

Once sufficiently cooked season to taste and ladle the hot stew into the mason jars. Be sure to leave one inch of headspace free.

Allow to cool and place lid on the jar.

Beef and Cheddar Mason Jar Salad

Not only is this salad tasty and nutritious for you it is fairly easy to make! It's great for a person who is on the go. Unless you wish for a marinated salad put the dressing on the bottom.

These salads can be safely stored for five days inside your refrigerator.

Ingredients

- Five quart sized mason jars
- Ten tablespoons thousand island yogurt dressing
- One quart cherry tomatoes, halved
- Five baby cucumbers, sliced and halved
- One half Spanish onion, diced
- Five single serving packets of cheddar cheese, chopped into cubes
- One half pound thinly sliced roast beef, chopped up
- Three cups spinach/arugula blend

Instructions

Divide all the ingredients among each mason jar. Pour the dressing into the mason jar first. This is done to prevent everything else from getting soggy. Next, add the tomatoes, and then the cucumbers, onion, cheese, roast beef, and finally the spinach/arugula.

Place the lid on the mason jar and seal it tightly. When you're ready to eat your salad you can give it a good shake and mix the ingredients around with your fork and you're set!

Steak Salad in a Jar

Do you like the above recipe but want to try something different? Why not add fruit? Fruit is a tasty addition to just about any salad. Unless you wish for a marinated salad put the dressing on the bottom.

Ingredients

- Ranch dressing
- Sliced carrots
- Cherry tomatoes
- Strawberries
- Blueberries
- Grass fed steak (sliced)
- Baby Romaine Salad
- Grated Swiss
- One quart mason jar

Instructions

Divide all the ingredients among each mason jar. Pour the ranch dressing into the mason jar first.

Next, add the carrots, and on top of those layer the tomatoes, strawberries, blueberries, steak, Baby Romaine Salad, and top with the layer of grated Swiss cheese.

Place the lid on the mason jar and seal it tightly. When you're ready to eat your salad you can give it a good shake and mix the ingredients around with your fork and you're set!

Chili in a Jar

Chili can be quite tasty for lunch. Now you can make your own chili to enjoy at any day!

For this recipe you will need a pressure canner.

Ingredients

- Three pounds ground beef
- Twenty four Roma tomatoes, peeled, seeded, and chopped (or 2 quarts canned tomatoes)
- Three cups dried beans, cooked and drained. Pinto or black beans work well.
- Two medium onions, chopped
- Two green, red, or yellow sweet peppers, seeded and chopped
- Two jalapeno peppers, diced
- Two cayenne peppers, diced
- Two teaspoons cumin
- One teaspoon salt
- Two teaspoons chili powder

- One teaspoon garlic powder

- One tablespoon cocoa powder

- Nine pint canning jars

Instructions

In a skillet brown the ground beef with an onion. Add the seasonings, cooked beans, peppers, and tomatoes. You can reduce or increase the amount of chili powder and hot peppers depending on how spicy you like your chili. Cook until the vegetables are tender.

You may need to add a little water or tomato juice into the mixture so the chili is not too thick for pressure canning. You'll want the chili to be a little runny.

Ladle into pint jars and wipe the rims.

Screw on the canning lids and process in the pressure canner for seventy five minutes at fifteen pounds pressure.

Chapter 3 – Mouth Watering Seafood Lunch Recipes

If you enjoy seafood here are four recipes that will not only satisfy your seafood cravings but will be great tasting!

Shrimp in a Jar

If you enjoy shrimp or have some extra shrimp around use them for this great recipe!

Ingredients

- Two medium tomatoes, chopped
- One fourth cup chopped white onion
- One fourth cup finely chopped cilantro or parsley
- One to two teaspoons chopped fresh jalapeno
- Two tablespoons ketchup
- Two to three tablespoons fresh lime juice, divided

- One pound peeled cooked shrimp, cut into one half inch pieces

- Two firm ripe avocados

- Two cups shredded lettuce

- One half cup coarsely crumbled tortilla chips

Instructions

In a bowl stir together tomatoes, onion, parsley, chili, ketchup, one tablespoon lime juice, and one half tea spoon salt.

Once stirred add shrimp and season to taste with salt and pepper.

Mash the avocados with the remaining one to two tablespoons of lime juice and one half teaspoon of salt.

Divide the lettuce among the jars and layer the shrimp mixture and avocado mixture. Top with the crumbled chips.

Asian Shrimp, Pineapple and Peanut Salad

If you still want to experiment with shrimp but want to try something different this is a great recipe to try!

Ingredients

Dressing:

- Two tablespoons fresh lime juice
- Two tablespoons fish sauce (for example, nam pla or nuoc nam)
- Two tablespoons olive oil
- One tablespoon sugar
- One half cup thinly sliced shallots
- One small jalapeño chili, thinly sliced
- Three tablespoons fresh mint leaves

Salad:

- Sixteen peeled deveined cooked large shrimp with tails intact
- Six ounces fresh pineapple, peeled, cut into two and one fourth inch spears

- One large avocado, halved, pitted, peeled, coarsely chopped

- Two tablespoons salted peanuts

- One lime, cut into eight wedges (for garnish)

Instructions

Dressing:

Whisk lime juice, fish sauce, oil, and sugar in a small bowl until the sugar dissolves. Stir in the shallots, chili, and mint.

Salad:

Toss shrimp with salt and pepper in a bowl. Add pineapple, avocado, and dressing.

Carefully place the salad and dressing into mason jars. Top with nuts and garnish with the lime wedges. Place the lids on and put the jars in the fridge.

Seafood Louie Salad

Here's something that is tasty with just about any type of seafood. Unless you wish for a marinated salad put the dressing on the bottom.

Ingredients

- One tablespoon low fat Thousand Island dressing

- One third cup cherry tomatoes

- One fourth cup celery chopped

- One hard-boiled egg, sliced

- One eighth avocado, diced

- Two tablespoons sliced black olives

- One third cup your favorite seafood. Crab, shrimp, etc.

- One and one half cups torn romaine lettuce

- One quart mason jar

Instructions

Add the low fat dressing to the bottom of your mason jar. On top of that place the chopped celery, and then the cherry tomatoes. Next, add your seafood, olives, hardboiled egg, and then the avocado. Top with the lettuce.

Place the lid on the jar and place inside your refrigerator. The salad should keep for five days.

Seafood Gnocchi in a Jar

If you like Seafood Gnocchi here's an easy and great tasting recipe to try!

Ingredients

- One fourth can Campbell's New England clam chowder soup

- One half can of tuna in water (drained)

- Gnocchi

- Salt

- Pepper

- Olive oil

- Four cherry tomatoes

- One half onion

- Provolone cheese

Instructions

In a skillet sauté the onion via your preferred method. Once tender remove from the skillet and set to the side.

Cook the Gnocchi in olive oil. Season to taste with the salt and pepper.

Inside the mason jar first pour in the New England clam chowder. On top of the clam chowder add the tuna, then the gnocchi, cherry tomatoes, onion, and top with the cheese.

Place the lid on the jar and seal tightly.

When you are ready to eat your meal remove the cheese and microwave the remaining contents for three minutes or until hot. Place the cheese back on top and you're set!

Chapter 4 – The Perfect Pork Lunch Time Recipes

Would you like to try some tasty pork lunch time recipes? Some of these may take a little time to make but are well worth the effort as you'll want to try them time and time again.

BBQ in a Jar

If you're food of BBQ this is a very tasty way to have some for lunch! You might want to have some paper plates around as BBQ can get messy.

Ingredients

- One cup plus two teaspoons table salt
- One half cup plus two tablespoons sugar
- One boneless pork butt (5 pounds will do you), cut in half horizontally so it's only half as thick. Store bought will do if you don't have enough time to make pulled pork.

- Two tablespoons ground black pepper
- Two tablespoons paprika
- One teaspoon cayenne pepper
- Your favorite BBQ sauce
- Your favorite baked beans
- Coleslaw
- Meat thermometer (only necessary if making your own pulled pork)

Instructions

Making the pulled pork: please note, if you are using store bought pulled pork please disregard this section. Instructions on layering the meal are below.

You will want to brine the pork seven hours before you need it. Get your biggest pitcher or bowl and fill it with water. Add and dissolve one cup salt and one half cup sugar. Place the pork in the mixture, cover, and let it sit for two hours.

While the pork, water, and sugar mixture sits, in a separate bowl, combine the black pepper, paprika, two tablespoons sugar, two teaspoons salt, and cayenne and set aside.

Preheat your oven to 325.

After the two hours have passed it's time to roast the pork. Remove the pork from the water, salt, and sugar mixture. Pat dry with paper towels.

Taking the back of a spoon rub the pre-made spices all over the surface of the pork.

Place the pork on a wire rack and set inside a foil-lined baking sheet. Cover the pork with aluminum foil and seal the edges so moisture doesn't escape.

Roast for three hours.

After three hours have passed remove the foil and roast the pork for another hour to an hour and a half. The internal temperature should be around 200 degrees F on the meat thermometer. Once fully cooked remove the pork from the oven and shred it with two forks. Add your favorite BBQ sauce and mix well so it's fully covered.

Layering

After all that work now comes the easy part of layering!

Start by adding the baked beans to the bottom of the mason jar. It's up to you to how much you wish to add. Next add the coleslaw and top with the pulled pork.

Frittata in a Jar

This delicious meal is great for lunch and easy to make. This is as tasty cold as it is warm and is quite nutritious.

Ingredients

- One half pound pork or four pieces of bacon
- One half bunch of kale, chopped
- One half red bell pepper, chopped
- Seven large eggs
- Two cups plain yogurt
- One half teaspoon salt

Instructions

Preheat your oven to 400 degrees F.

While your oven warms up start cooking the pork into a pan and break it up into small pieces until cooked through. If you are using bacon fry it until it is crispy and then chop it into small pieces. Once cooked remove from the pan and drain the fat and liquids and return the meat to the pan.

Add the red bell pepper and cook for three minutes.

Next add the kale and cook until it has wilted.

In a large bowl beat the eggs and add the yogurt and salt. Beat this mixture until it is well mixed.

Divide the meat and vegetable mixture into six one half pint mason jars.

Top the jars off with the egg mixture and leave one inch head space.

Place the jars on a cookie sheet and place into the oven. Let bake for twenty five to thirty minutes or until the mixture is set and golden on top.

Saucy Pulled Pork Cornbread Muffins

Cornbread being cooked inside mason jars may seem a little silly at first but the idea is quickly gaining momentum as people come up with their own delicious and creative ideas. For this recipe you will want a smaller mason jar.

These pulled pork cornbread muffins are easy to make and easy to take with you.

Ingredients

- One cup fine yellow cornmeal
- One and one half cups flour
- Four teaspoons sugar
- Four teaspoons baking powder
- One half teaspoon salt
- One and one fourth cup milk
- Two eggs
- One third cup canola oil
- One cup pulled pork
- Your favorite barbecue sauce
- Small pickles or slices of pickle (optional)

Instructions

Preheat oven to 375 degrees F.

Prepare your small mason jars by using your favorite non-stick baking spray.

In a large bowl combine the cornmeal, flour, sugar, baking powder, and salt.

In another bowl mix together your milk, eggs, and oil.

Pour the wet ingredients into the dry and beat until well mixed and smooth.

Divide about two thirds of the batter among the prepared mason jars. Add a generous teaspoon of the pulled pork in the middle of each jar. Top with the remaining batter and leave about one inch of headspace.

If you're adding a pickle garnish now is the time to do so. Bake for 20-25 minutes.

Smokey Dry-Rubbed Pork Tenderloin Apple and Dijon Mustard Salad in a Jar

This is a great way to switch up a traditional salad and try something new! How many vegetables, salad greens, mustard, apple butter, and mayonnaise you add is up to you.

Ingredients

- Dry rub for pork
- One small pork tenderloin chop
- Mayonnaise
- Apple butter
- Dijon mustard
- One mason jar
- Vegetables (carrots, cabbage, etc.)
- Salad greens of your choice

Instructions

Preheat your broiler on high for ten minutes.

Coat the pork chops in dry rub and flatten by hitting the meat with the palm of your hand onto a hard surface.

Place the pork chops on a baking sheet and place in the oven until it is browned and the fat is crisped. Turn the pork chop over and let it brown. This only takes a few minutes so you will want to keep a close eye on them.

Inside your mason jar first add the sliced pork chop followed by the mayonnaise, apple butter, and mustard. Now use your heavy veggies such as carrots, shredded cabbage, etc. On top of that add your light vegetables such as your salad greens.

Chapter 5 – Quick & Easy Vegetarian Lunch Recipes

After all those recipes about meat I don't want anyone who is vegetarian or considering the vegetarian diet to think I have forgotten about you. I truly haven't! Below are four tasty and healthy vegetarian style mason jar lunch recipes for you to try and enjoy.

Fresh corn, edamame, and radish salad

Here's a tasty salad that has tasty vegetables that you may even be able to grow in your own back yard!

Ingredients

- Two cups fresh corn
- Two cups shelled edamame
- One cup chopped radishes
- Two tablespoons chopped green onion
- Two tablespoons chopped cilantro
- One fourth cup canola oil

- Two tablespoons rice vinegar

- Two teaspoons white miso paste

- Two teaspoons chili garlic sauce (optional)

Instructions

Combine your corn, edamame, radishes, green onion, and cilantro in a large bowl and mix well.

In another bowl whisk together the canola oil, rice vinegar, white miso paste, and chili garlic sauce.

Pour the dressing mixture into the greens mixture and toss well.

Divide into mason jars and place the lids in place. Place these jars in your refrigerator and let refrigerate for at least an hour.

Before eating be sure to give the mason jar a good shake.

Chunky Mediterranean Mason jar salad

If you enjoy Mediterranean food or wish to try it for the first time this is a great place to start! The recipe involves cheese, but if you are not open for consuming dairy it can be skipped and you can still have a great new salad to try! Unless you wish for a marinated salad put the dressing on the bottom.

Ingredients

Eight tablespoons red wine vinaigrette

Two cups red sugar plum tomatoes

Two cups chopped English cucumber

Two cups pitted Kalamata olives

Two cups fired-roasted red and yellow peppers, thinly sliced

Two cups red onion, chopped

Two cups crumbled feta cheese (optional)

Instructions

Inside a large mason jar pour in the vinaigrette first. On top of that add your plum tomatoes followed by the English cucumber, olives, peppers, onion, and top with the feta cheese.

Place the lid on your mason jar and let it sit in your refrigerator until you're ready to eat it.

Be sure to shake the jar well when you are ready to eat your salad.

Field Berry Salad

Do you feel like something with fruit as well as vegetables? Here's a delicious and simple salad to try that should more than satisfy those needs! Unless you wish for a marinated salad put the dressing on the bottom.

Ingredients

- Red wine vinegar
- Shredded carrots
- Red onion, sliced thinly
- Blueberries
- Mandarin oranges
- Sliced almonds
- Arugula

Instructions

Inside a large mason jar pour in the vinegar first. On top of the vinegar add your carrots, onion, blueberries, mandarin oranges, and arugula. Top with the slice almonds.

Place the lid on your mason jar and let it sit in your refrigerator until you're ready to eat it.

Be sure to shake the jar well when you are ready to eat your salad.

Asian Salad

Here's another healthy vegetarian friendly salad. It's a great way to expand your palate and get to try new foods and ideas. Unless you wish for a marinated salad put the dressing on the bottom.

Ingredients

- Annie's shiitake sesame vinaigrette dressing
- Shredded carrots
- Diced cucumbers
- Sprouts
- Red bell pepper, diced
- Mandarin oranges (patted dry)
- Edamame
- Mixed baby greens
- Sesame seeds

Instructions

Inside a large mason jar pour in the Annie's shiitake sesame vinaigrette dressing first. On top of the vinaigrette add the shredded carrots, edamame, mixed baby greens, red bell pepper, diced cucumber, mandarin oranges, sprouts, and then the greens. Top with sesame seeds.

Place the lid on your mason jar and let it sit in your refrigerator until you're ready to eat it.

Be sure to shake the jar well when you are ready to eat your salad.

Your Mason Jar Lunches Journey

Thank you again for downloading this book! I hope you enjoyed all the delicious mason jar lunch recipes I've included. Why spend money on eating out when you can make your own tasty lunches at a fraction of the price?

So now I have taken you on a journey into the world of mason jar meals, I really hope this book will help benefit you, your friends and families health and wellbeing.

The next step is to take action on what you have learned today. I'm sure with the right practice and listening to my directions step by step of the way you will become a mason jar pro in no time!

Be sure to look out for my other Mason Jar meals book I've wrote with include daily meals and amazing mason jar salads.

Finally, if you enjoyed this book, then I'd like to ask you for a favor, would you be kind enough to leave a review for this book on Amazon? It'd be greatly appreciated!

Bon Apetite,

Kathy Hunt

)

Mason Jar Salads

Quick and Easy Salads On The Go

By Kathy Hunt

Contents

Introduction

Welcome to this beginners recipe guide on the beauty of using mason jar salads, where you will discover how to whip up the most amazing mason jar salads which will save you time and money, but most of all better your overall health.

If you have never experienced using mason jar meals, then you will be blown away with what you will discover inside this quick and easy jar salads book.

Inside I will teach you the little known tips and tricks to get the best results from your mason jar salads which will save you hours of time trying to figure it out on your own.

Enjoy!

Kathy Hunt

Chapter 1 – The Setup for Mason Jar Salads

Mason jar meals are gaining popularity among all sorts of people. Despite the appearance these salads have they are relatively simple and easy to make. You won't have to worry about any sort of "fail" or the dreaded "nailed it!" joke that accompanies an odd looking item.

These are great things to make as you can make them up to a week in advance for your lunches or other meals. Making them will also save you time and money!

Does making a salad feel like a monstrous task? There are unlimited options for making salads and mason jar salads are no different. They are simply on a smaller scale and in mason jars.

To make a mason jar salad the one thing you definitely need is a mason jar! These can be bought in bulk for a fairly inexpensive price or may even by lying around at home. Quite often it's recommended to get them in the quart size. If a quart is too big you can always scale down.

You may need bowls, whisks, forks, spoons, pots and pans, and skillets along with other basic kitchen utensils.

Some people prefer to use wide mouthed funnels when making mason jar meals. You can purchase wide mouthed funnels for often a very inexpensive price at your local grocery store.

Making mason jar meals is a fairly easy process that just about anyone can do. If you can layer items you can make a mason jar salad!

When you plan to make some of your mason jar salads make sure that your kitchen is clean. Wash out your mason jars with warm soapy water and let them dry.

Be sure to clean your fruits and vegetables via your preferred method. If you have to cut them up into pieces you can do so now which will save you time later.

You'll want to have lids that fit your jars. Screw on lids are often the best type.

Some recipes will call for you to leave the full mason jar inside the refrigerator for a few hours to allow to chill or for the flavors to blend. These can often be made a few days in advance and allowed to sit inside the refrigerator.

Most mason jar salads will last for seven days before starting to spoil. If you aren't certain about how long the salad will last you can check the life span of the vegetables or fruits you have put inside your mason jar.

Some people like to get creative and like to vacuum seal their mason jars once they are full. This is not a necessary step, but if you want to do so to remove any excess moisture or air you are free to do so. Vacuum sealing your mason jars will not harm the contents inside or damage the jars. Many of these seals can be bought at your grocery store or at a canning store for a good price.

Chapter 2 – Layering Your Salad with The Key Ingredients in Your Jars

Generally you can put all sorts of things inside a mason jar.

When it comes to mason jar salads the most important thing is layering. Unless you want a marinade or the recipe calls for it, you will want to put your dressing down at the very bottom.

The next thing you'll be adding are the hard vegetables that won't soak up the dressing. These hard vegetables can include tomatoes, radishes, peas, and other vegetables.

After the hard vegetables are added, there may be more "softer" vegetables or fruits that will be layered. These can include corn, onions, cucumbers, and other vegetables and fruits.

On the very top of the salad will be the greens such as lettuce or cabbage.

On this layer of lettuce people may also add cheese or seeds.

If you aren't certain about which layer goes where, there are many mason jar salad recipes that will list what order you layer each item in.

The more tightly you pack your salad the less air there will be inside the mason jar. The less air there is the better tasting and fresher it will be.

To help get everything good and mixed when they are ready to eat, many people prefer to give their mason jar a good shake. If that's not an option, you can pour the contents into a good sized bowl and give it a good stir to get everything blended.

Some people prefer to bring a salad bowl with them when they eat their mason jar salad. Others are content with eating straight from the jar so which method you choose is entirely up to you.

Chapter 3 – My Top Tasty Mason Jar Salad Recipes

Are you ready to try some tasty and healthy for you salads? There is no limit to what types of salads you can create in mason jars! Be sure to have fun and even create your own creative salads and ideas!

Unless you prefer a marinade salad or the recipe calls for it it's best to put any dressing first so it's at the bottom of the mason jar.

Canned Cobb Salad

This is a healthy and delicious take on a salad that is very easy to make.

Ingredients

Dressing:

- One tablespoon Greek yogurt
- One half teaspoon mayo
- One teaspoon mustard
- One eighth teaspoon honey

Salad

- One fourth cup shredded carrot

- One fourth cup cooked peas

- Two tablespoons minced onion

- Three tablespoons broccoli, chopped, florets only

- Two slices bacon, chopped

- One hard-boiled egg, chopped

- One tablespoon sunflower seeds

- One and one half cup romaine lettuce, chopped

Instructions

In a bowl whisk the ingredients for the dressing. Once it has been well mixed carefully pour the contents into your mason jar.

Next, layer the cooked peas, followed by the carrots, broccoli, onion, hard-boiled eggs, bacon, and top with the lettuce and sunflower seeds.

Tex-Mex Salad

This hearty recipe contains plenty of veggies and meat that will help keep you full and give you some of the greens and meats you need in your diet.

Ingredients

- Two teaspoons balsamic vinegar
- One tablespoon salsa
- One fourth cup bell pepper, diced
- One third cup shredded chicken
- One fourth cup cooked corn
- One fourth cup black beans
- Two tablespoons cheese
- One tablespoon olives, sliced
- Two and one half cups romaine lettuce, chopped

Instructions

Mix the balsamic vinegar and salsa together. With a spoon carefully ladle them to the bottom of your mason jar.

Next, layer the chicken followed by the corn, black beans, olives, cheese, pepper, and top with the lettuce.

Japanese Salad

If you like the taste of Japanese food or wish to try a Japanese salad now is the perfect time to do so with this recipe!

Ingredients

Dressing

- One tablespoon white miso paste
- One tablespoon water
- One teaspoon rice vinegar
- One teaspoon sugar
- One half teaspoon peanut butter
- One eighth teaspoon sesame oil

Salad

- One half cup chicken
- One fourth cup thinly sliced bell pepper
- Two tablespoons pickled daikon and carrot
- Three tablespoons edamame beans, cooked

- One fourth cup sliced cucumber

- Two tablespoons green onion (white and light green parts only)

- One half cup thinly sliced cabbage

- One and one half cups romaine lettuce

Instructions

In a bowl whisk together the ingredients for the dressing until smooth. Carefully ladle into a mason jar.

On top of the dressing layer the chicken, pickled daikon and carrot, edamame beans, cucumber, onion, bell pepper, and top with the cabbage and lettuce.

This salad will keep for two days so be sure to eat it soon!

Ranch Rotini Salad

If you have any left-over noodles or dressing this is a great way to use them and to make for a tasty salad.

Ingredients

- Two tablespoons ranch dressing

- One cup al dente cooked rotini pasta, cooled

- One fourth of one small bunch broccoli florets, cut into bite size pieces

- One tablespoon diced red onion

- One half of an celery stalk, diced

- Three grape tomatoes

- One ounce cubed smoked cheddar cheese

Instructions

Pour the ranch dressing into your mason jar first. On top of the dressing layer in the pasta, broccoli, red onion, celery, grape tomatoes, and top with the cheese.

Salad shaker

Do you prefer a smaller salad or something that you can eat quickly? The salad shaker is here for you! This is a salad that only takes minutes to prepare.

Ingredients

- Two tablespoons balsamic vinaigrette dressing

- Three fresh white mushrooms, sliced

- Five cherry tomatoes

- One cup fresh spinach leaves, stems removed

Instructions

Pour the balsamic vinaigrette in first. Next add the mushrooms, cherry tomatoes, and top with the spinach. Give the jar a good shake when you're ready to eat and you are good to go!

Spring Vegetable Orzo Pasta Salad

If you enjoy asparagus and artichokes this is a wonderful salad to make!

Ingredients

- One bunch asparagus, about three cups diced

- One tablespoon olive oil

- Two shallots, minced

- Two cloves garlic, minced

- Twelve ounces orzo pasta, cooked to al dente and cooled

- Fifteen ounce can artichoke hearts

- One and one half cups sun-dried tomatoes in olive oil

- One lemon, zested and juiced

- One fourth cup white wine vinegar

- One teaspoon kosher salt

- One half teaspoon fresh ground black pepper

- One third cup olive oil

Instructions

Fill a medium sauce pan full of water and bring to a boil. Once the water is boiling turn off the burner and add in the asparagus pieces and let sit for two to three minutes.

While the asparagus is in the water heat one tablespoon olive oil in a small sauté pan. Next add in the shallots and garlic and sauté for one to two minutes. They should be just tender.

Once the asparagus is ready drain it and rinse with cool water.

In a large bowl add the cooked orzo pasta, asparagus pieces, the sautéed shallots, and the garlic. Drain the artichoke hearts and quarter them before adding them to the bowl. Add in the sun-dried tomatoes and the oil and lemon zest. Stir this mixture well to combine.

In a small bowl whisk together the lemon juice, white wine vinegar, salt, and pepper. Continue to whisk the mixture as you slowly pour the olive oil into the vinegar. Once it has been well mixed add the dressing to the salad.

Carefully ladle your salad into the mason jars and place the lids on them. Place the mason jars into the refrigerator for at least five hours so the flavors can combine.

Fiesta Quinoa Salad

This salad is great for those who are vegetarian, can't have gluten, or are lactose intolerant. It is also a very healthy recipe and tastes great.

Ingredients

- One cup quinoa
- One tablespoon olive oil
- One medium onion, chopped
- Three garlic cloves, minced
- Two cups water
- One half teaspoon kosher salt
- One half teaspoon ground black pepper

Dressing

- One teaspoon olive oil
- One teaspoon white wine vinegar
- One eighth teaspoon kosher salt
- One teaspoon taco seasoning
- One half teaspoon ground chia seeds (optional)

Salad

- One fourth cup corn (fresh or frozen); patted dry if wet

- One fourth cup black beans, rinsed, drained, and patted dry

- One teaspoon diced jalapeno

- Six to eight small grape or cherry tomatoes, left whole (optional)

- One cup packed greens (optional); cut romaine lettuce, uncut arugula, uncut baby spinach, or shredded cabbage

Instructions

In a strainer rinse the quinoa under running water for at least sixty seconds. Once the water runs clear you can drain it.

In a two quart pan on your stove top heat the olive oil over medium-high heat. Add the onions and cook until soft. Add the garlic and stir for one minute. Next add the water, quinoa, salt, and pepper. Bring the mixture to a boil and then lower the heat. Cover the pan and let simmer for fifteen minutes. After fifteen minutes have passed remove the pan from the heat, remove the lid, and fluff with a fork. Set the pan aside and allow to cool completely.

Combine the dressing ingredients in a bowl and stir them well with a fork or a whisk. Once well mixed carefully pour the dressing into the bottom of your mason jar. Add one half cup of the cooked and cooled quinoa pilaf and use a fork to toss with the dressing until well mixed.

On top of the quinoa and dressing mixture layer the corn, black beans, jalapenos, cherry tomatoes, and top with the greens.

Pasta Salad

Here's a unique salad to try if you're a fan of pasta!

Ingredients

- Two ounces Italian dressing
- One fourth onions, chopped
- One half green pepper, chopped
- One half red pepper, chopped
- One fourth black olives, sliced
- Pepperoni to your liking
- Two ounces cooked pasta

Instructions

Pour the Italian dressing into the bottom of the mason jar. Next, add the onions, green peppers, red peppers, and black olives. Add the pepperoni and top with the cooked pasta.

When you're ready to eat give the jar a good shake and you're ready to go.

Caprese Pasta Salad

Here's another delicious Italian salad to try!

Ingredients

- Four ounces balsamic vinaigrette

- One cup cherry tomatoes

- One and one half ounce fresh Mozzarella, cut into bite size pieces

- Two ounces cooked penne pasta

- One half cup spinach leaves

- One half cup fresh basil, chopped

Instructions

Pour the dressing into the bottom of the mason jar. Next add the cherry tomatoes followed by the penne pasta. Top this with the mozzarella pieces and top with the spinach and basil.

Chef Salad

Have you ever wanted to try a chef salad? There's no time like the present to start with this tasty recipe!

Ingredients

- Four ounces dressing of your choice
- One half cup carrot matchsticks
- One fourth black olives, sliced
- One fourth cup diced cucumber
- One fourth diced tomato
- One fourth green and/or red pepper
- One fourth chopped ham and/or turkey
- One to two hard-boiled eggs, diced
- Lettuce, variety of choice

Instructions

Pour the dressing onto the bottom of your mason jar. Next layer the carrot matchsticks, black olives, cucumber, tomato, green/red pepper, meat, eggs, and top with the lettuce.

Greek Salad with Chickpeas and Feta

If you like Greek salad this is a great one to try! You can also make it in under fifteen minutes. This is also wonderful for vegetarians and is filled with protein.

Ingredients

- Two ripe tomatoes, chopped
- One English cucumber, chopped
- Two bell peppers, seeded and chopped
- One red onion, diced
- One fourteen ounce can of no salt added chickpeas, rinsed and drained
- One cup of light feta or goat feta
- One tablespoon extra-virgin olive oil
- Two tablespoons lemon juice
- One fourth teaspoon dried oregano
- Salt and pepper to taste

Instructions

Whisk together the olive oil, lemon juice, oregano, salt, and pepper in a small bowl. Once well blended carefully pour the dressing into the bottom of the jar.

On top of the dressing layer the tomatoes, cucumber, bell peppers, onion, chickpeas, feta, and top with the lettuce.

Fresh and Springy Walnut, Radish, and Apple Salad

Here's a great salad if you wish to add some fruits, nuts, and get your veggies in at the same time!

Ingredients

- Three tablespoons raw almond butter
- One tablespoon unseasoned rice wine vinegar
- One eighth teaspoon salt
- One tablespoon maple syrup
- Two teaspoons toasted sesame oil
- Three cups mixed greens
- 1 stalk celery, diced
- Two to three radishes, thinly sliced
- One fourth green apple, thinly sliced and soaked in salted water to prevent browning
- One third cup walnuts

Instructions

In a bowl combine the raw almond butter, rice wine vinegar, salt, maple syrup, and the sesame oil. Stir well until well blended. Once mixed carefully spoon two tablespoons of the mixture into the bottom of your mason jar.

Next layer the apples, radishes, celery, and walnuts. Top with the greens and seal your jar. Place in the refrigerator until you are ready to eat.

Burrito Bowl salads

If you enjoy chipotle this is a wonderful recipe to try!

Ingredients

Quinoa

- One cup quinoa

- Two cups water

- One half teaspoon salt

- Juice and zest of one lime

- One fourth cup chopped fresh cilantro

Chicken

- Two large chicken breasts

- Two teaspoons sea salt

- One tablespoon coconut oil or ghee

Sweet potatoes

One large sweet potato, washed and with both ends cut off

One tablespoon residual bacon oil or coconut oil

Other

- Three cups chopped lettuce

- Five tablespoons Greek yogurt

- Three fourths cup shredded cheese

- One half cup chopped fresh cilantro

- Two strips thick cut bacon (optional)

Instructions

Quinoa

Add the quinoa, water, and salt into a medium sized pot. Bring to a boil over medium heat. When it has reached a boil cover and cook for twenty to twenty-five minutes or until the quinoa is soft and fluffy.

Once this is done remove the pot from the heat and set the quinoa aside to cool.

Once it has cooled add the lime juice, lime zest, and one fourth cup chopped cilantro to the rice and stir. You can add more lime and cilantro as needed according to taste.

Chicken

Dry both chicken breasts with paper towels. Season both sides of each breast with two teaspoons of salt.

In a large skillet heat one tablespoon coconut oil over a medium-high heat until the oil is quite hot.

Add both the chicken breasts to the hot skillet and cook for about four minutes on each side.

Once the chicken breasts are cooked remove them from the skillet and place them on a cutting board to cool. Once they've cooled cut the chicken into small chunks no more than one half inch square.

Bacon

If you wish to add bacon in your salad cook two slices of bacon via your preferred method until it is crispy enough to crumble. Save one tablespoon of bacon fat for the sweet potatoes and drain and discard of the rest.

Sweet potatoes

Cut the sweet potato into small pieces about one half square inch wide.

Heat one tablespoon of bacon fat (if you didn't use bacon, use coconut oil instead) in a large skillet over medium heat.

When the oil is hot add the sweet potato cubes. Sear the potatoes on all sides by stirring every three to five minutes.

When the potatoes have browned on the outside turn the heat down to medium-low and cover the skillet with a lid. Cook the sweet potatoes until they can easily bee pierced with a fork. When this has happened set them aside to cool.

Assembly

When all the ingredients have cooled you can assemble the burrito bowl salads.

Add one tablespoon of Greek yogurt to the bottom of each mason jar. Next add two tablespoons of sweet potato cubes, followed by three to four tablespoons of the cilantro lime quinoa, one to two tablespoons of cheese, bacon, chicken, and top with lettuce. If you wish you can sprinkle some chopped cilantro before screwing on the lid.

Zucchini Noodle Salad with Peas and Quinoa

This is a great recipe that is as protein packed as it is tasty!

Ingredients

Dressing

- One half of an avocado
- Two tablespoons coconut milk
- Juice from half of one lime

Salad

- One third cup cooked quinoa
- Two teaspoons minced cilantro
- One and one half teaspoon coconut flakes
- Three asparagus stalks, chopped into one inch pieces
- One fourth cup green peas
- One medium zucchini
- Two to three scallion stalks, diced
- One fourth cup cubed feta

Instructions

In a bowl or a blender mix all the ingredients for the dressing until creamy and set aside.

In a bowl combine the quinoa, cilantro, and coconut flakes. Toss them to combine and set aside.

Fill a small sauce pan half way with water and bring to a boil. Add the asparagus and one minute later add the peas. Cook for three to four minutes or until the vegetables are fully cooked.

Add the dressing to the mason jar first. Upon that layer the zucchini noodles, quinoa, scallions, asparagus and peas, and then the feta.

Place the lid on your mason jar and then place in the refrigerator.

Asian Noodle Salad

If you've ever wished to try an Asian noodle salad now is the best time to try it! This tasty salad has a nice "kick" to it which makes it very tasty.

Ingredients

Spicy peanut dressing

- Two tablespoons peanut butter
- Four teaspoons sambal oelek
- Four teaspoons rice vinegar
- Four teaspoons soy sauce
- One fourth cup extra virgin olive oil
- One tablespoon black sesame seeds

Salad

- Four ounces soba noodles
- One red bell pepper, thinly sliced
- One cup shelled edamame, cooked
- Two large carrots, peeled and shredded
- Four green onions, thinly sliced
- One half cup crunchy rice noodles

Instructions

Fill a large pot with water and bring to a boil and cook the noodles according to the package instructions.

While the noodles cook it's time to make the spicy peanut dressing. In a small bowl whisk together the peanut butter, sambal oelek, rice vinegar and soy sauce. While whisking slowly add in the oil and add the sesame seeds.

Divide the spicy peanut dressing among four pint sized mason jars. Next add the soba noodles to each jar. On top of that layer the remaining ingredients and end with the rice needles. Add the lid to the mason jar and place inside the refrigerator. The salads will last for five days.

Mason Jar Salads Conclusion

Thank you again for downloading this book! I hope you've enjoyed reading about all the great mason jar salad recipes available for you to try.

Make sure you also check out my other mason jar meals books which are always full of fresh new ideas to help you benefits from this tasty way of life.

The next step is to take action on what you have learned today. I'm sure with the right practice and listening to my directions step by step of the way you will become a mason jar pro in no time!

Finally, if you enjoyed this book, then I'd like to ask you for a favor, would you be kind enough to leave a review for this book on Amazon? It'd be greatly appreciated!

Bon Apetite,

Kathy Hunt